AFFIRMATIONS FOR DARK SKINNED TEENS:

Discovering and Empowering One's Inner self

James Stones

TABLE OF CONTENT

Introduction

Embark on a transformative journey of self-discovery with this empowering guide! Within these pages, we invite you, our vibrant readers, to explore the compelling impact of affirmations. This book is more than just words; it's a celebration of your identity, a roadmap to cultivate unwavering confidence, and a guide to navigating the unique challenges you may face. Let's together unlock your inner strength, embrace your heritage, and affirm the incredible potential within each of you. Are you ready to commence a journey of self-love, triumph, and limitless possibilities? Join us as we begin this inspiring odyssey!

Welcoming Words

Greetings and a warm embrace to you, dear reader! As you delve into the heart of this book, consider this not just a guide but a companion on your quest for personal growth and empowerment. Within these pages, we embark on a shared exploration of the power of affirmations—a journey tailor-made for the vibrant souls seeking to navigate the intricate tapestry of identity, confidence, and resilience.

Here, the welcome extends beyond mere words; it's an invitation to join a community, a collective of individuals eager to celebrate the richness of their heritage and the boundless potential within. This isn't just a book; it's a sanctuary where affirmations become the keys to unlocking the doors of self-love and triumph.

As you navigate through each chapter, envision this as a conversation between kindred spirits—one that acknowledges the unique challenges you may face, celebrates your triumphs, and provides the tools to build unshakeable confidence. So, with open hearts and eager minds, let's embark on this odyssey together, where words become affirmations, and affirmations transform lives. Welcome to a transformative journey—one that begins with you.

The Power of Affirmations

Within the fabric of self-discovery, affirmations emerge as dynamic threads weaving a narrative of empowerment. Beyond simple words, they act as agents of transformation, possessing the power to shape thoughts and carve destinies. This chapter unravels the core of affirmations—their capacity to transcend the ordinary and propel individuals toward a realm where self-belief stands as the bedrock of success.

Envision affirmations as gentle whispers of encouragement, resonating through the corridors of your mind, guiding you toward self-love, confidence, and triumph. As we navigate the intricacies of these positive declarations, we uncover the secret language that speaks directly to the subconscious, fostering a mindset that embraces possibilities and overcomes challenges.

Embark on a journey where words cease to be mere expressions, transforming into tools for personal growth. Within the realm of affirmations, discover the untapped reservoir of strength within you, eagerly waiting for acknowledgment and activation. Welcome to the exploration of "The Power of Affirmations," where each phrase carries the potential to reshape your reality.

Chapter 2

Identity and Pride

In the vibrant tapestry of your personal odyssey, the inaugural chapter unfurls as a jubilant fête dedicated to "Identity and Pride." Here, we extend an invitation to fully immerse yourself in the profound significance of your distinctive identity—a narrative intricately woven with the opulent threads of heritage and culture.

Visualize this chapter as a compass, a guiding force orchestrating your journey through the landscapes of self-discovery. It beckons you to revel in the splendor of your roots, recognizing the fortitude embedded in the intricate weave of your heritage. The affirmations bestowed within this chapter transcend beyond mere words; they metamorphose into powerful expressions of self-love, spinning a tale that connects your past, empowers your present, and foreshadows a resilient future.

As you plunge into the exploration of identity, envisage these affirmations as mirrors, each reflecting the quintessence of your true self. Let this chapter be a sanctum, a sacred space where you unearth the beauty in every strand of your identity—a jubilant celebration of your essence, a declaration of pride that radiates from embracing your unique self.

Embark on this voyage of self-discovery, where "Identity and Pride" intertwine to paint the canvas of your narrative with vivid hues. May the affirmations within this chapter harmonize with the pulsating rhythm of your heart, fostering an unshakable pride in your identity—a pride that resounds with authenticity, strength, and the unbridled richness of your unique story.

Embracing Black Excellence

In the expansive realm of personal growth, the ensuing chapter unfolds as an exuberant exploration into "Embracing Black Excellence." Consider this segment as an immersive journey, a call to fully embrace and revel in the richness of your black identity—a celebration of excellence that transcends societal narratives.

Envision this chapter as a tapestry woven with threads of accomplishment and resilience. It beckons you to immerse yourself in the narratives of black excellence, where affirmations serve as empowering mantras that echo the achievements, the triumphs, and the limitless potential within. These affirmations are not just words; they metamorphose into beacons of inspiration, lighting the path toward recognizing and embracing the extraordinary capabilities inherent in the black experience.

As you navigate the landscape of this chapter, visualize affirmations as brushstrokes on a canvas, crafting a portrait of Black Excellence that goes beyond stereotypes and challenges societal norms. This is a celebration of your unique talents, a testament to the resilience embedded in the black experience, and a declaration of the unbounded potential awaiting realization.

Embark on this odyssey, where "Embracing Black Excellence" becomes a journey of self-affirmation, self-celebration, and a bold assertion of the brilliance ingrained in your identity. May the affirmations within this chapter resonate as a chorus of empowerment, inspiring you to recognize, embrace, and showcase the extraordinary tapestry of Black Excellence that defines your narrative.

Affirmations for SelfLove and Heritage

In the expansive realm of self-discovery, the following chapter gracefully unfolds as a poetic exploration titled "Affirmations for Self-Love and Heritage." Picture this segment as an enchanting journey, an invitation to immerse yourself in the intricacies of affirmations that intricately weave together the threads of self-love and heritage, crafting a narrative that is uniquely yours.

Imagine this chapter as a haven, a sacred space where affirmations transcend mere words to become potent elixirs, nurturing the seeds of self-love and cultural pride. Each affirmation echoes the resonance of your heritage, resembling melodic notes that serve as a constant reminder of the strength ingrained in your identity. These affirmations take the form of love letters to oneself, expressed in the language of affirmation, fostering a deep connection between your heart and the rich tapestry of your cultural roots.

As you navigate through the verses of this chapter, visualize affirmations as brushes delicately painting strokes of self-love onto the canvas of your soul. This chapter is an ode to the inherent beauty within, a recognition of the profound value that accompanies the embrace of your heritage.

Affirmations, in this context, transform into a ritual—
a daily practice that not only nurtures self-love but
also pays homage to the legacy of those who
paved the way.

Embark on this poetic sojourn, where "Affirmations
for Self-Love and Heritage" metamorphose into
verses composing the anthem of your identity. May
these affirmations resonate as harmonies, weaving
a narrative that blends the melody of self-love with
the rich chords of heritage, creating a symphony
that joyously celebrates the beauty inherent in
every facet of your being.

Chapter 3

Confidence Unleashed

In the expansive tapestry of personal growth, the ensuing chapter gracefully unveils itself as an exploration entitled "Confidence Unleashed." Envision this section as a captivating odyssey, an invitation to immerse yourself in the nuanced journey of unlocking and embracing boundless confidence, a journey uniquely tailored for your empowerment.

Consider this chapter a sanctuary, a space where affirmations cease to be mere words, metamorphosing into catalysts that unfurl the wings of confidence within you. Each affirmation resonates as a powerful declaration, a beacon that guides you through the labyrinth of self-doubt and societal expectations, unlocking the reservoirs of unwavering self-assurance.

As you traverse the verses of this chapter, visualize affirmations as keys, each unlocking a door to a realm where stereotypes are shattered, and confidence is no longer confined by limitations. This is an anthem of self-empowerment, a chorus that reverberates with the understanding that your unique qualities are strengths, not shortcomings.

Embark on this odyssey, where "Confidence Unleashed" becomes a transformative journey, a narrative where affirmations breathe life into the dormant seeds of self-assurance. May these affirmations echo as declarations, resonating with the melody of your individuality, and heralding the emergence of a confident, empowered version of yourself.

Breaking Stereotypes

In the grand tapestry of self-exploration, the forthcoming chapter gently reveals itself as an expansive odyssey entitled "Breaking Stereotypes." Envision this segment as an immersive sojourn, a heartfelt invitation to embark on a transformative expedition dedicated to dismantling entrenched preconceptions and boldly rewriting narratives that have long sought to confine and constrain.

This chapter unfolds as a sanctuary, a sacred space where affirmations cease to be mere utterances and metamorphose into formidable agents of change. Each affirmation stands as a formidable force, a potent instrument meticulously designed to dismantle the restrictive walls of stereotypes that have persistently impeded the full expression of your unique identity.

As you traverse the verses of this chapter, visualize affirmations as skillful chisels meticulously sculpting a liberating path, where stereotypes crumble under the weight of authenticity. This is a resounding declaration of emancipation from societal expectations, an anthem that boldly champions the inherent beauty found in embracing your distinctive qualities, which defy and challenge conventional norms.

Embark on this profound odyssey, where "Breaking Stereotypes" evolves into a narrative of significance, a symphony of affirmations that resonates with the harmonious rhythm of authenticity. May these affirmations resound as powerful declarations, not merely breaking down barriers but completely transforming the landscape, paving the way for a narrative that is unapologetically, authentically, and beautifully yours.

Affirmations for Unshakeable Confidence

In the vast expanse of personal growth, the ensuing chapter elegantly reveals itself as a captivating journey titled "Affirmations for Unshakable Confidence." Picture this segment as an immersive odyssey, an invitation to traverse the landscapes of self-assurance with affirmations that serve as steadfast companions, guiding you toward the pinnacle of unyielding confidence.

Imagine this chapter as a haven, a sacred space where affirmations cease to be mere words and evolve into potent elixirs, fortifying the foundations of your self-assurance. Each affirmation resonates as a powerful decree, a beacon illuminating the path to unwavering confidence amidst life's ebbs and flows.

As you navigate the verses of this chapter, visualize affirmations as pillars supporting the edifice of your self-esteem, unyielding in the face of doubt and uncertainty. This is a symphony of self-empowerment, where affirmations become affirmations of resilience, echoing with the understanding that your confidence is not dependent on external validations but arises from the wellspring of self-belief within.

Embark on this transformative odyssey, where "Affirmations for Unshakable Confidence" becomes a narrative of significance, a symphony of declarations that resonate with the harmonious rhythm of self-assurance. May these affirmations echo as powerful affirmations, instilling in you a confidence so unshakeable that it becomes the bedrock upon which you navigate the journey of life with resilience and unwavering certainty.

Chapter 4

Triumph over Challenges

In the expansive tapestry of personal evolution, the subsequent chapter gracefully unravels itself as a profound expedition entitled "Triumph Over Challenges." Picture this segment as a poignant odyssey, an invitation to immerse yourself in the transformative journey of not just confronting but conquering the myriad challenges that life presents.

Envision this chapter as a sanctuary, a space where affirmations cease to be mere utterances and metamorphose into resilient mantras, navigating you through the complex terrain of challenges. Each affirmation stands as a resolute companion, a guiding light that not only acknowledges the hurdles but propels you toward victorious outcomes.

As you traverse the verses of this chapter, visualize affirmations as arrows in your quiver, each meticulously aimed at overcoming obstacles with precision and fortitude. This is a symphony of triumph, where affirmations become affirmations of resilience, echoing with the understanding that challenges are not roadblocks but opportunities for growth and transformation.

Embark on this poignant odyssey, where "Triumph Over Challenges" becomes a narrative of resilience, a symphony of declarations that resonate with the harmonious rhythm of victory. May these affirmations echo as powerful affirmations, instilling in you the fortitude to face challenges head-on, turning adversity into stepping stones toward personal growth and triumph.

Confronting Racism

In the expansive tapestry of personal growth, the following chapter unfolds as a poignant exploration titled "Confronting Racism." Envision this segment as a profound odyssey, an invitation to delve into the transformative journey of not merely acknowledging but actively challenging and dismantling the complex layers of racism that persist in our society.

Consider this chapter a sanctuary, a space where affirmations cease to be mere words and evolve into powerful instruments of change, guiding you through the intricate and often challenging terrain of confronting racism. Each affirmation becomes a courageous declaration, a beacon illuminating the path toward fostering understanding, dismantling biases, and advocating for equality.

As you navigate the verses of this chapter, visualize affirmations as seeds planted in the soil of consciousness, each one contributing to the growth of empathy, compassion, and a collective commitment to eradicating racism. This is a symphony of activism, where affirmations become affirmations of resilience, echoing with the understanding that the journey towards dismantling racism is not only a personal endeavor but a collective responsibility.

Embark on this transformative odyssey, where "Confronting Racism" becomes a narrative of societal change, a symphony of declarations that resonate with the harmonious rhythm of advocacy and justice. May these affirmations echo as powerful affirmations, instilling in you the courage and determination to contribute to the broader movement towards a more inclusive, equitable, and anti-racist society.

Resilience in the Face of Obstacles

In the vast expanse of personal development, the subsequent chapter gracefully unfolds as an enlightening exploration titled "Resilience in the Face of Obstacles." Envision this segment as a profound odyssey, an invitation to immerse yourself in the transformative journey of not just encountering but triumphing over the diverse and formidable obstacles that life presents.

Consider this chapter as a sanctuary, a space where affirmations cease to be mere expressions and evolve into potent tools for resilience, guiding you through the intricate terrain of facing and overcoming obstacles. Each affirmation stands as a resolute companion, a guiding light that not only acknowledges the challenges but empowers you to navigate them with unwavering strength and tenacity.

As you traverse the verses of this chapter, visualize affirmations as stepping stones on your path, each strategically placed to bolster your resilience and fortitude. This is a symphony of triumph, where affirmations become affirmations of empowerment, echoing with the understanding that obstacles are not barriers but opportunities for growth and transformation.

Embark on this enlightening odyssey, where "Resilience in the Face of Obstacles" becomes a narrative of personal strength, a symphony of declarations that resonate with the harmonious rhythm of overcoming adversity. May these affirmations echo as powerful affirmations, instilling in you the resilience to face obstacles head-on, turning challenges into catalysts for profound personal growth and triumph.

Chapter 5

Flourishing Relationships

In the expansive tapestry of personal growth, the subsequent chapter gracefully unveils itself as a heartfelt exploration titled "Flourishing Relationships." Envision this segment as a captivating odyssey, an invitation to immerse yourself in the transformative journey of nurturing and cultivating relationships that not only endure but thrive.

Consider this chapter as a haven, a sanctuary where affirmations cease to be mere expressions and metamorphose into powerful tools for building and sustaining flourishing relationships. Each affirmation becomes a guiding principle, a beacon illuminating the path towards deep connections, understanding, and shared growth.

As you traverse the verses of this chapter, visualize affirmations as seeds sown in the fertile soil of connection, each one contributing to the blossoming of love, trust, and mutual support. This is a symphony of unity, where affirmations become affirmations of harmony, echoing with the understanding that flourishing relationships are not static but dynamic, evolving through communication, empathy, and shared experiences.

Embark on this captivating odyssey, where "Flourishing Relationships" becomes a narrative of meaningful connections, a symphony of declarations that resonate with the harmonious rhythm of mutual growth and support. May these affirmations echo as powerful affirmations, inspiring you to invest in the richness of your relationships, creating a tapestry of love and understanding that stands the test of time.

Building Positive Bonds

In the vast realm of personal development, the ensuing chapter gracefully unfolds as a profound exploration titled "Building Positive Bonds." Envision this segment as an enriching odyssey, an invitation to immerse yourself in the transformative journey of intentionally fostering and nurturing positive connections that serve as pillars of support and growth.

Consider this chapter as a sanctuary, a space where affirmations transcend mere utterances and transform into robust tools for the intentional cultivation of positive bonds. Each affirmation becomes a guiding principle, a beacon illuminating the path towards the construction of meaningful relationships that uplift, inspire, and withstand the tests of time.

As you traverse the verses of this chapter, visualize affirmations as the foundation stones in the construction of positive bonds, each one contributing to the resilience and depth of your connections. This is a symphony of unity, where affirmations evolve into affirmations of shared values, echoing with the understanding that positive bonds flourish through communication, empathy, and a shared commitment to mutual well-being.

Embark on this enriching odyssey, where "Building Positive Bonds" becomes a narrative of intentional connections, a symphony of declarations that resonate with the harmonious rhythm of shared growth and support. May these affirmations echo as powerful affirmations, inspiring you to invest in the richness of your relationships, fostering a network of positive bonds that elevate and empower both you and those with whom you share these meaningful connections.

Affirmations for Family and Friendship

In the vast canvas of personal development, the forthcoming chapter unfolds as an intricate exploration titled "Affirmations for Family and Friendship." Envision this segment as a profound odyssey, an invitation to immerse yourself in the transformative journey of fostering affirmations that not only strengthen familial bonds but also deepen the tapestry of friendship.

Consider this chapter a sanctuary, a sacred space where affirmations cease to be mere words and metamorphose into powerful expressions designed to nurture the essence of family and friendship. Each affirmation becomes a guiding light, illuminating the path toward building resilient connections, fostering understanding, and cultivating a shared journey of growth.

As you traverse the verses of this chapter, visualize affirmations as seeds sown in the fertile soil of relationships, each one contributing to the flourishing of familial love and the blossoming of enduring friendships. This is a symphony of unity, where affirmations become declarations of mutual support, echoing with the understanding that family and friendship are dynamic bonds requiring intentional care, communication, and a shared commitment to each other's well-being.

Embark on this profound odyssey, where "Affirmations for Family and Friendship" becomes a narrative of meaningful connections, a symphony of declarations that resonate with the harmonious rhythm of shared growth, support, and the enduring strength of bonds that withstand the test of time. May these affirmations echo as powerful expressions, inspiring you to nurture and cherish the richness of your familial and friendly connections, creating a tapestry of love, understanding, and enduring camaraderie.

Chapter 6

Academic Mastery

In the expansive tapestry of personal and intellectual growth, the ensuing chapter elegantly reveals itself as a profound exploration titled "Academic Mastery." Envision this segment as a scholarly odyssey, an invitation to immerse yourself in the transformative journey of not merely navigating academic pursuits but mastering the art of learning, understanding, and excelling in your educational endeavors.

Consider this chapter a haven, a sacred space where affirmations cease to be mere expressions and metamorphose into powerful tools for cultivating academic excellence. Each affirmation becomes a guiding principle, a beacon illuminating the path toward embracing the challenges of education with resilience, curiosity, and an unwavering commitment to intellectual growth.

As you traverse the verses of this chapter, visualize affirmations as the ink that inscribes your educational narrative, each one contributing to the flourishing of knowledge, critical thinking, and a profound understanding of your academic pursuits. This is a symphony of learning, where affirmations become declarations of academic prowess, echoing with the understanding that mastering one's educational journey involves diligence, passion, and a thirst for continuous learning.

Embark on this scholarly odyssey, where "Academic Mastery" becomes a narrative of intellectual prowess, a symphony of declarations that resonate with the harmonious rhythm of educational achievement. May these affirmations echo as powerful expressions, inspiring you to approach your academic endeavors with confidence, dedication, and a fervent desire to not only succeed but thrive in the pursuit of knowledge and academic excellence.

Excelling in Education

Within the expansive realm of personal and academic growth, the following chapter gracefully unveils itself as an enlightening exploration titled "Excelling in Education." Envision this segment as an educational odyssey, an invitation to immerse yourself in the transformative journey of not only navigating the academic landscape but mastering the intricacies of learning, understanding, and achieving excellence in your educational pursuits.

Consider this chapter a sanctuary, a sacred space where affirmations transcend mere expressions and metamorphose into potent tools for cultivating academic brilliance. Each affirmation stands as a guiding principle, a beacon illuminating the path toward embracing the challenges of education with resilience, curiosity, and an unwavering commitment to intellectual growth.

As you traverse the verses of this chapter, visualize affirmations as the ink that inscribes your educational narrative, each one contributing to the flourishing of knowledge, critical thinking, and a profound understanding of your academic pursuits. This is a symphony of learning, where affirmations become declarations of scholarly prowess, echoing with the understanding that excelling in education involves diligence, passion, and a continual thirst for knowledge.

Embark on this enlightening odyssey, where "Excelling in Education" becomes a narrative of intellectual mastery, a symphony of declarations that resonate with the harmonious rhythm of educational achievement. May these affirmations echo as powerful expressions, inspiring you to approach your academic journey with confidence, dedication, and an unwavering commitment to not only succeed but to truly thrive in the pursuit of knowledge and academic excellence.

Affirmations for Academic Success and Goal Pursuit

In the expansive journey of personal and academic growth, the subsequent chapter gracefully unfurls as an empowering exploration titled "Affirmations for Academic Success and Goal Pursuit." Envision this segment as a scholarly odyssey, an invitation to immerse yourself in the transformative journey of not just achieving academic success but also navigating the intricate path of setting and realizing educational goals.

Consider this chapter a haven, a sacred space where affirmations cease to be mere expressions and metamorphose into potent tools for cultivating not only academic excellence but also a roadmap for goal pursuit. Each affirmation becomes a guiding star, illuminating the path toward embracing the challenges of education, setting ambitious goals, and navigating the academic journey with resilience, curiosity, and an unwavering commitment to success.

As you traverse the verses of this chapter, visualize affirmations as the ink that inscribes your educational narrative, each one contributing to the flourishing of knowledge, critical thinking, and a profound understanding of your academic pursuits. This is a symphony of learning, where affirmations become declarations of scholarly prowess, echoing with the understanding that academic success and goal pursuit involve diligence, passion, and a continual thirst for knowledge.

Embark on this empowering odyssey, where "Affirmations for Academic Success and Goal Pursuit" becomes a narrative of intellectual mastery and achievement, a symphony of declarations that resonate with the harmonious rhythm of educational success and the fulfillment of ambitious aspirations. May these affirmations echo as powerful expressions, inspiring you to approach your academic and goal-setting endeavors with confidence, dedication, and an unwavering commitment to not only succeed but to truly thrive in the pursuit of knowledge and personal achievement.

Chapter 7

Nurturing Mental WellBeing

In the expansive tapestry of personal well-being, the forthcoming chapter gracefully unveils itself as a profound exploration titled "Nurturing Mental Well-Being." Envision this segment as a compassionate odyssey, an invitation to immerse yourself in the transformative journey of not only acknowledging but actively nurturing the intricate landscape of your mental health.

Consider this chapter a sanctuary, a sacred space where affirmations cease to be mere expressions and metamorphose into powerful tools for cultivating a resilient and flourishing mental state. Each affirmation becomes a guiding light, illuminating the path toward embracing self-care, fostering emotional resilience, and navigating the complexities of mental well-being with compassion, self-awareness, and a commitment to inner peace.

As you traverse the verses of this chapter, visualize affirmations as seeds planted in the fertile soil of your consciousness, each one contributing to the blossoming of mindfulness, self-compassion, and a profound understanding of your mental and emotional states. This is a symphony of self-care, where affirmations become declarations of personal growth, echoing with the understanding that nurturing mental well-being is a continuous journey involving self-love, acceptance, and intentional mindfulness.

Embark on this compassionate odyssey, where "Nurturing Mental Well-Being" becomes a narrative of self-care and emotional resilience, a symphony of declarations that resonate with the harmonious rhythm of inner peace and holistic well-being. May these affirmations echo as powerful expressions, inspiring you to approach your mental health with gentleness, mindfulness, and a steadfast commitment to cultivating a thriving and resilient state of mind.

Stress Management

In the intricate tapestry of personal well-being, the subsequent chapter gracefully unfolds as an insightful exploration titled "Stress Management." Envision this segment as a guiding compass, an invitation to immerse yourself in the transformative journey of not merely confronting but actively managing the complex and often challenging facets of stress.

Consider this chapter a sanctuary, a space where affirmations become powerful tools for cultivating resilience and navigating the ebbs and flows of stress with grace and intention. Each affirmation stands as a guiding principle, a beacon illuminating the path toward embracing stress as a natural part of life while equipping yourself with strategies to mitigate its impact.

As you traverse the verses of this chapter, visualize affirmations as anchors, grounding you in moments of turbulence and uncertainty. This is a symphony of self-care, where affirmations become declarations of empowerment, echoing with the understanding that stress management involves intentional choices, self-compassion, and a commitment to your well-being.

Embark on this insightful odyssey, where "Stress Management" becomes a narrative of personal empowerment, a symphony of declarations that resonate with the harmonious rhythm of resilience and balance. May these affirmations echo as powerful expressions, inspiring you to approach stress with a mindful perspective, fostering a resilient mindset, and cultivating a harmonious equilibrium in the face of life's challenges.

Mindfulness Affirmations

In the expansive realm of personal well-being, the ensuing chapter gracefully reveals itself as an enlightening exploration titled "Mindfulness Affirmations." Picture this segment as a serene journey, an invitation to immerse yourself in the transformative practice of not only acknowledging but actively cultivating mindfulness in every facet of your life.

Consider this chapter a sanctuary, a sacred space where affirmations cease to be mere expressions and transform into potent tools for nurturing present-moment awareness, tranquility, and a deep connection with the essence of each moment. Each affirmation becomes a guiding whisper, leading you toward a mindful state where you embrace the richness of your experiences, fostering a heightened sense of clarity, calmness, and appreciation.

As you traverse the verses of this chapter, visualize affirmations as seeds of awareness planted in the fertile soil of your consciousness, each one contributing to the flourishing garden of mindfulness. This is a symphony of self-discovery, where affirmations become declarations of being fully present, echoing with the understanding that mindfulness is a journey of intentional living, self-compassion, and an unwavering commitment to the beauty inherent in each breath.

Embark on this enlightening odyssey, where "Mindfulness Affirmations" becomes a narrative of self-awareness and tranquility, a symphony of declarations that resonate with the harmonious rhythm of a mindful and fulfilling life. May these affirmations echo as powerful expressions, inspiring you to approach each moment with mindfulness, fostering a deep connection with yourself and the world around you.

Chapter 8

Paving the Path to the Future

In the grand tapestry of personal growth, the subsequent chapter gracefully unveils itself as an expansive exploration titled "Paving the Path to the Future." Envision this segment as a visionary odyssey, an invitation to immerse yourself in the transformative journey of not only envisioning but actively crafting the trajectory that will lead you toward a future rich with purpose, fulfillment, and achievement.

Consider this chapter a sanctuary, a space where affirmations cease to be mere expressions and metamorphose into powerful tools for setting intentions, cultivating resilience, and navigating the path to the future with clarity and purpose. Each affirmation becomes a guiding star, illuminating the way toward the realization of your aspirations, the fulfillment of your potential, and the creation of a future that aligns with your deepest values.

As you traverse the verses of this chapter, visualize affirmations as building blocks, each contributing to the construction of a foundation that supports your goals and aspirations. This is a symphony of self-discovery and intentional living, where affirmations become declarations of purpose, echoing with the understanding that paving the path to the future involves deliberate choices, continuous growth, and a steadfast commitment to the journey ahead.

Embark on this visionary odyssey, where "Paving the Path to the Future" becomes a narrative of intentional living, a symphony of declarations that resonate with the harmonious rhythm of purposeful endeavors and the shaping of a future that reflects the very essence of your aspirations. May these affirmations echo as powerful expressions, inspiring you to actively participate in the creation of a future that aligns with your vision, values, and the fulfillment of your true potential.

Career Dreams and Aspirations

In the expansive journey of personal and professional development, the ensuing chapter elegantly reveals itself as an illuminating exploration titled "Career Dreams and Aspirations." Envision this segment as a visionary odyssey, an invitation to immerse yourself in the transformative journey of not merely harboring but actively pursuing and realizing the aspirations that shape your professional path.

Consider this chapter a sanctuary, a sacred space where affirmations cease to be mere expressions and metamorphose into powerful tools for envisioning, planning, and navigating the intricate landscape of your career dreams. Each affirmation becomes a guiding beacon, illuminating the way toward the fulfillment of your professional potential, the realization of your career aspirations, and the creation of a meaningful and purpose-driven professional trajectory.

As you traverse the verses of this chapter, visualize affirmations as building blocks, each contributing to the construction of a foundation that supports your career goals and dreams. This is a symphony of intentional career development, where affirmations become declarations of purpose, echoing with the understanding that cultivating a fulfilling professional journey involves deliberate choices, continuous growth, and a steadfast commitment to the pursuit of your career aspirations.

Embark on this visionary odyssey, where "Career Dreams and Aspirations" becomes a narrative of intentional professional growth, a symphony of declarations that resonate with the harmonious rhythm of purposeful endeavors and the shaping of a career that aligns with the very essence of your aspirations. May these affirmations echo as powerful expressions, inspiring you to actively pursue and manifest the career of your dreams, embracing the opportunities and challenges that come with the fulfillment of your professional potential.

Making a Positive Impact

In the vast canvas of personal growth and societal contribution, the subsequent chapter gracefully unfolds as a profound exploration titled "Making a Positive Impact." Picture this segment as an altruistic odyssey, an invitation to immerse yourself in the transformative journey of not only recognizing but actively cultivating opportunities to leave a lasting, positive imprint on the world around you.

Consider this chapter a sanctuary, a space where affirmations cease to be mere expressions and metamorphose into powerful instruments for promoting positive change, compassion, and the betterment of society. Each affirmation becomes a guiding principle, a beacon illuminating the way toward creating meaningful impact, fostering kindness, and contributing to a world that reflects the values of empathy and positive transformation.

As you traverse the verses of this chapter, visualize affirmations as seeds planted in the fertile soil of societal well-being, each one contributing to the flourishing garden of positive change. This is a symphony of altruism, where affirmations become declarations of purpose, echoing with the understanding that making a positive impact involves intentional choices, empathy, and a steadfast commitment to the betterment of the world.

Embark on this altruistic odyssey, where "Making a Positive Impact" becomes a narrative of intentional contribution, a symphony of declarations that resonate with the harmonious rhythm of societal betterment. May these affirmations echo as powerful expressions, inspiring you to actively seek opportunities for positive impact, fostering a legacy of kindness, compassion, and meaningful change in the lives of others and the world at large.

Conclusion (Harmony Within)

In the culmination of this transformative journey, the concluding chapter elegantly emerges as a reflective exploration titled "Harmony Within." Envision this segment as a poignant culmination, an invitation to immerse yourself in the integration of the affirmations, insights, and lessons learned throughout this profound odyssey.

Consider this chapter a sanctuary, a space where the echoes of affirmations resonate with the harmonious rhythm of your inner self. Each reflection becomes a guiding light, illuminating the path toward a balanced and harmonious existence, where the integration of newfound perspectives fosters personal growth, resilience, and a deep sense of fulfillment.

As you traverse the verses of this concluding chapter, visualize affirmations as the threads weaving together the tapestry of your personal journey. This is a symphony of self-discovery and integration, where the culmination of affirmations becomes a declaration of the harmony achieved within, echoing with the understanding that personal growth is an ongoing process of embracing the journey with compassion, self-awareness, and a commitment to living a harmonious life.

Embark on this reflective odyssey, where "Harmony Within" becomes a narrative of self-realization, a symphony of declarations that resonate with the harmonious rhythm of personal balance and fulfillment. May these affirmations echo as powerful expressions, inspiring you to embrace the harmonious essence within, fostering a life of authenticity, purpose, and the continual pursuit of personal harmony.

Reflections and Encouragement

In the closing stages of this transformative exploration, the concluding chapter gracefully unfolds as a contemplative journey titled "Reflections and Encouragement." Picture this segment as a reflective sanctuary, an invitation to immerse yourself in the transformative process of contemplating the affirmations, insights, and the profound growth experienced throughout this odyssey.

Consider this chapter as a sacred space, where affirmations cease to be mere expressions and metamorphose into echoes of encouragement, guiding you to reflect on the profound lessons learned and the strides made in personal and emotional development. Each reflection becomes a guiding beacon, illuminating the path toward self-awareness, resilience, and a heartfelt encouragement to continue embracing the journey with authenticity and determination.

As you traverse the verses of this concluding chapter, visualize affirmations as echoes of encouragement, resonating with the harmonious rhythm of your evolving self. This is a symphony of self-discovery, where the reflections become declarations of resilience, echoing with the understanding that personal growth is a continuous journey requiring self-compassion, self-awareness, and a steadfast commitment to one's own well-being.

Embark on this contemplative odyssey, where "Reflections and Encouragement" becomes a narrative of self-affirmation, a symphony of declarations that resonate with the harmonious rhythm of personal empowerment and encouragement. May these reflections echo as powerful expressions, inspiring you to continue your journey with newfound determination, authenticity, and an unwavering commitment to your ongoing growth and well-being.

Navigating Your Affirmation Journey

In the expansive narrative of personal growth, the subsequent chapter gracefully unveils itself as a comprehensive exploration titled "Navigating Your Affirmation Journey." Envision this segment as a strategic map, an invitation to immerse yourself in the transformative process of not only embracing but actively navigating the intricate terrain of your affirmation journey.

Consider this chapter a guide, a sanctuary where affirmations cease to be mere expressions and transform into dynamic tools for personal navigation, growth, and empowerment. Each affirmation becomes a marker on your journey, illuminating the path toward self-discovery, resilience, and the realization of your aspirations.

As you traverse the verses of this chapter, visualize affirmations as milestones, each contributing to the unfolding narrative of your personal evolution. This is a symphony of intentional living, where affirmations become declarations of purpose, echoing with the understanding that charting your affirmation journey involves deliberate choices, continuous self-reflection, and a steadfast commitment to your ongoing well-being.

Embark on this strategic odyssey, where "Navigating Your Affirmation Journey" becomes a narrative of intentional personal growth, a symphony of declarations that resonate with the harmonious rhythm of empowerment and the shaping of a life that aligns with your deepest values and aspirations. May these affirmations echo as powerful expressions, inspiring you to actively navigate your affirmation journey with purpose, resilience, and a commitment to the continuous exploration and realization of your true potential.

Affirmation Treasury

In the closing chapters of this transformative odyssey, the final segment gracefully unfolds as an enriching exploration titled "Affirmation Treasury." Envision this section as a treasure trove, an invitation to immerse yourself in the transformative wealth of affirmations accumulated throughout this profound journey.

Consider this chapter a sanctuary, a sacred space where affirmations cease to be mere expressions and metamorphose into valuable gems of wisdom, each carrying the essence of personal growth, resilience, and self-discovery. Each affirmation becomes a precious coin in the treasury, contributing to the richness of your emotional and mental wealth.

As you traverse the verses of this concluding chapter, visualize affirmations as treasures, each holding the power to inspire, uplift, and guide you on your ongoing journey. This is a symphony of self-discovery, where the treasury becomes a testament to the transformative power of affirmations, echoing with the understanding that personal growth is a continuous process, and the treasury serves as a timeless resource for empowerment.

Embark on this enriching odyssey, where the "Affirmation Treasury" becomes a narrative of accumulated wisdom, a symphony of declarations that resonate with the harmonious rhythm of self-affirmation and continual well-being. May these affirmations echo as precious expressions, inspiring you to return to this treasury whenever needed, drawing upon the wealth of wisdom and empowerment it holds for your ongoing journey of personal growth.

A Compilation of Empowering Affirmations

In the profound anthology of personal empowerment, envision this compilation as a symphony of affirmations, each note resonating with the power to inspire, uplift, and ignite transformative change. As you delve into these affirmations, let them not merely be words but guiding beacons, illuminating the path to your inner strength, resilience, and the unwavering belief in your limitless potential.

Affirmation of Self-Belief:
In the sanctuary of my being, I hold an unshakeable belief in my abilities and the boundless potential within me. Today, I embrace the power of self-belief as the driving force propelling me toward my dreams.

Courageous Resilience:
In the face of challenges, I stand resilient, like a sturdy oak weathering life's storms. I draw strength from adversity, transforming challenges into stepping stones toward my greatest achievements.

Radiant Self-Love:
Within me resides a boundless well of self-love. I embrace my flaws and celebrate my uniqueness, recognizing that my journey is a canvas painted with the vibrant colors of self-acceptance.

Manifesting Abundance:
I am a magnet for prosperity, abundance, and positive energy. My thoughts align with the abundant universe, and I attract the wealth of opportunities and success that is rightfully mine.

Unleashing Creativity:
My mind is a boundless wellspring of creativity. I embrace my unique ideas and express them fearlessly, contributing my creative essence to the world with confidence and authenticity.

Harmony in Relationships:
In the dance of connections, I cultivate harmony and understanding. I nurture relationships that uplift and support, creating a tapestry of love, trust, and shared growth.

Academic Mastery and Continuous Learning:
With each challenge, I embrace the opportunity to learn and grow. My academic journey is a canvas of continuous exploration, where knowledge and understanding unfold with each step.

Mindful Presence:

I am fully present in this moment, embracing the beauty of now. Mindfulness guides my actions, fostering clarity, peace, and a profound connection with the present.

Positive Impact:

My actions ripple with positive impact. I contribute to the betterment of the world, fostering kindness, compassion, and positive change in the lives of those around me.

Paving the Future:

I am the architect of my future. With purposeful intention, I carve a path toward success, fulfillment, and the actualization of my dreams.

May these affirmations resonate within you, weaving a tapestry of empowerment that accompanies you on your journey, inspiring greatness, and nurturing the realization of your true potential.

**GO OUT THERE AND MAKE US PROUD
I'M ROOTING FOR YOU.**

www.ingramcontent.com/pod-product-compliance
Lightning Source LLC
Chambersburg PA
CBHW060812260726
48660CB00002B/909

* 9 7 9 8 8 7 7 2 0 8 7 7 3 *